SNUFF OUT DIABETES TYPE 2

Wellness Redefined: unique strategies to Reverse Type 2 Diabetes and Thrive" "

Bridget F Brummit Phd

Copyright

All rights reserved. This publication may not be distributed or transmitted in any form or by any means, including photocopying, recording, or other electronic or mechanical methods, without prior written permission from the publisher. The only exceptions are brief quotations included in critical viewpoints and other noncommercial uses allowed by copyright law.

Disclaimer

Information in book "SNUFF OUT DIABETES TYPE 2" is intended only for general education use. Although every attempt has been made in good faith by the author and publisher to present accurate and current content, they neither explicitly represent nor guarantee that the information contained herein is reliable, accurate, appropriate, complete, or available.

Both the author and the publisher do not accept responsibility for any loss or harm that arises from using the material in the book.

Table of contents

Table of Contents

CHAPTER 1

Permit me to introduce you to my mother an Experienced endocrinologist her name is Dr. Jessica Brummit.

She had a shocking turn in her health when she learned she had type 2 diabetes. The irony of her circumstances struck her, and she made the decision to treat her illness with the same commitment and skill that she had shown her patients for years.

Well-known for her thorough research, Dr. Jessica Brummit examined the most recent findings and developments in the treatment of diabetes. Equipped with this knowledge, she created a customized treatment plan that combined clinical competence with doable lifestyle adjustments.

Dr. Jessica worked with a nutritionist to create a sustainable and well-balanced food plan because she recognized the importance of diet. She adopted a low-glycemic lifestyle, emphasizing fresh vegetables, lean meats, and good fats. One of the pillars of her patient care philosophy is the journey she took to rethink her relationship with food.

As a passionate supporter of physical exercise, Dr. Jessica led by example by included exercise in her daily regimen. She found the joy of movement and its beneficial effects on insulin sensitivity through everything from brisk walks to more intense workouts. Her newly discovered interest had an impact on her personal health as well as becoming a major topic of discussion when she spoke with patients.

Renowned for her empathetic approach to patient care, Dr. Jessica disclosed her personal diabetes diagnosis to patients during their visits. Through sharing her experiences, she developed a stronger connection and empathy with her patients. Her waiting room became a place where people could confide, offer counsel, and support one another.

Dr. Jessica started diabetes support groups because she understood the value of a strong sense of community. These events gave people a forum for discussing problems, exchanging helpful advice, and sharing success stories. Previously regarded as an authority, Dr. Jessica evolved into a confidante and mentor for people managing the complications of diabetes.

Dr. Jessica investigated mindfulness and stress reduction methods as part of her quest for holistic health. As useful techniques for managing her diabetes, she shared these practices with her patients and adopted them into her own life. Her clinic changed, becoming a place where patients could get complete support for their health in addition to medical advice.

Although there were challenges along the way for Dr. Jessica, her perseverance and dedication to preventive health management eventually produced favorable results. Her experience inspired patients and staff to face diabetes with hope and empowerment, and it reached beyond the walls of her clinic. By showing that one might traverse the path to wellness with knowledge, compassion, and a strong dedication to a balanced life, even in the face of unforeseen health issues,

I grew up so fond of my mother and this inspired my choice of the medical profession, as a mother and a professional colleague, so I choose to share this experience and proven methods that worked for my mother and my patients over the years to help other patients in this condition.

Set off on a life-changing path to improved health by buying "Snuff Out Diabetes Type 2."

This book is packed with useful tips for reviving your lifestyle, such as adopting energizing workout regimens and embracing delectable, diabetes-friendly cuisine. This book is filled to the brim with motivational tales, practical guidance, and a road map for taking back control of your wellbeing.

Elevated blood glucose, often known as blood sugar, is a defining feature of diabetes, a chronic metabolic disease that eventually causes major harm to the heart, blood vessels, eyes, kidneys, and nerves.

Diabetes is a complex metabolic disease characterized by the body's inability to control blood glucose levels. The main energy source for cells is glucose, which comes from the food we eat. The pancreas secretes the hormone insulin, which is essential for enabling cells to absorb glucose. Diabetes is caused by either insufficient insulin production by the pancreas or a decrease in the body's cells' sensitivity to the hormone's effects.

Traditional signs and symptoms include weight loss, thirst, polyuria, and impaired eyesight. If the illness is not treated, it may result in problems with the heart, kidneys, eyes, and nerves, among other health issues. An estimated 1.5 million fatalities annually result from diabetes that is either treated inadequately or untreated..

Approximately 422 million individuals globally suffer from diabetes, with the majority residing in low- and middle-income nations. The disease is the primary cause for 1.5 million fatalities annually. Over the past few decades, there has been a steady rise in both the number of cases and the incidence of diabetes.

Damage of blood arteries at both the macrovascular and microvascular levels is one of the main long-term consequences of diabetes. Cardiovascular disease increases the risk of diabetes, and coronary artery disease accounts for nearly 75% of diabetes-related deaths.Stroke and peripheral artery disease are two more macrovascular morbidities

Nerves, kidneys, and eyes are all impacted by microvascular illness. The most prevalent cause of blindness in those of working age is diabetic retinopathy, or damage to the retina. There are more conditions that might harm the eyes, such as glaucoma and cataract formation. Individuals with diabetes should see an ophthalmologist or optometrist once a year

More than half of American dialysis patients have diabetic nephropathy, which is a leading cause of chronic kidney disease. Nerve damage caused by diabetes can show up as a variety of symptoms, such as neuropathic pain, sensory loss, and autonomic dysfunction (which includes symptoms including erectile dysfunction, postural hypotension, and diarrhea). Lack of pain perception makes a person more vulnerable to injuries that can result in diabetic foot complications (such ulcers), which are the main cause of non-traumatic lower limb amputations.

There seems to be a possibility that type 2 diabetes and gallstones are related, based on a large body of evidence and multiple occurrences of gallstone disease. Compared to people without diabetes, those who have diabetes have an increased chance of gallstone development.

Research has indicated a connection between diabetes and cognitive impairment, with diabetics experiencing a higher risk and a faster pace of cognitive loss in comparison to people without the condition. Additionally, the illness increases the risk of falls in the elderly, particularly in those receiving insulin

Diabetes has its origins in prehistoric societies and is now recognized as a medical problem. Ancient manuscripts mentioned sweet-tasting urine, which suggested that the early observations in Egypt and India might have been signs of diabetes. The foundation for the eventual knowledge of the condition was established by these preliminary observations.

The medical community's knowledge of diabetes has progressively changed over time. Early attempts to define and describe diabetes were aided by the contributions of Greek and Roman physicians, including Aretaeus of Cappadocia. Yet it wasn't until the 20th century that diabetes was reduced from a deadly illness to a treatable one thanks to the crucial discovery of insulin.

The emergence of the industrial era resulted in notable changes to lifestyles, which were attributed to industrialization. Contemporary society has become characterized by urbanization, nutritional shifts, and decreased physical activity levels. Obesity and diabetes have been steadily rising as processed foods—which are heavy in sugar and bad fats—have become more common.

Dietary patterns have become more widely distributed since the 20th century. The increasing accessibility of processed foods and sugary beverages has made diets that were previously distinctive to a given region into a global commodity. The proliferation of food habits linked to a higher risk of diabetes was aided by globalization.

Disease patterns altered as nations moved from rural to industrial economies. Diabetes and other chronic illnesses started to replace infectious diseases, which had previously been prevalent. Changes in diet, lifestyle, and healthcare were reflected in this epidemiological shift.

The global obesity epidemic began in the last half of the 20th century. Since obesity and Type 2 diabetes are strongly related, obesity has grown to be a serious public health issue. Diabetes rates grew due in part to the obesity pandemic, which was fueled by sedentary lifestyles, higher calorie intake, and a lack of physical activity.

A rise in the prevalence of diabetes can be attributed to changes in the global population, particularly in regions where people are living longer. The increasing number of elderly people in the community has increased the burden of diabetes generally, as age is a major risk factor for Type 2 diabetes.

In addition, part of the diabetes epidemic was largely caused by socioeconomic issues. Diagnosis discrepancies in diabetes prevalence were partly caused by the difficulties that people from poorer socioeconomic backgrounds frequently had in getting access to healthcare, wholesome food, and physical exercise chances.

Sedentary Behaviors and Technological developments: In the late 20th and early 21st centuries, sedentary occupations and greater automation were brought about by technological developments. Physical activity levels have decreased, partly due to the emergence of digital technology and the popularity of screen-based entertainment.

Diabetes has become an international health concern, across country boundaries. The epidemic's global reach was facilitated by a number of factors, including expanding urbanization, shifting demographics, and the spread of bad lifestyle choices.

The diabetes epidemic is a result of the complex interactions between genetics, lifestyle, socioeconomics, and global dynamics, rather than being exclusively attributed to one issue. Diabetes is a complex global health issue that affects people of all ages, communities, and healthcare systems due to the convergence of various elements across time.

Overtime, diabetes has gone from being an uncommon condition to an epidemic. Many people are suffering, and sadly, despite their best efforts and substantial financial outlays,

the health authorities have given up and left the problem to worsen for the world's fastest-growing population. Ultimately declared type 2 diabetes to be a chronic, slowly fatal illness because they were unable to find a treatment.

Authorities have informed the majority of victims that they must rely on prescription drugs, medical equipment, and surgery to maintain their condition for the rest of their lives. But In this book our focus is on Diabetes type 2,

Diabetes can be in two forms namely;_

Type 1 Diabetes:

In Type 1 diabetes, the immune system attacks and kills the pancreatic beta cells that produce insulin by mistake. This autoimmune reaction causes a significant insulin shortage, which prevents cells from efficiently absorbing glucose.

Because of this, people with Type 1 diabetes require daily insulin injections or the use of an insulin pump in order to keep their blood sugar levels under control. Although type 1 diabetes is the most prevalent form identified in patients under the age of 20 and accounts for 5 to 10% of cases, the term "juvenile-onset diabetes" is no longer used because the disease frequently manifests as an adult.

The condition is defined by the death of the pancreatic islets' insulin-producing beta cells, which results in a severe insulin shortage. It is further divided into immune-mediated and idiopathic subtypes (where the etiology is unknown).

Most cases are immune-mediated, where an autoimmune onslaught driven by T cells results in beta cell death and consequently in insulin insufficiency. Patients frequently have blood sugar levels that are erratic and unpredictable as a result of extremely low insulin and a compromised ability to counteract hypoglycemia.

Type 1 diabetes is partially hereditary; the risk of the disease is known to be influenced by a number of genes, including specific HLA genotypes. Diabetes may develop in individuals who are genetically predisposed to the disease if one or more environmental variables, such as food or a virus, are present. Although a number of viruses have been linked, there is currently insufficient proof to back up this theory in human beings.

Any age can develop type 1 diabetes, however most cases are discovered in maturity. When type 1 diabetes strikes an adult, the condition is diagnosed as latent autoimmune diabetes of adults (LADA); it manifests later in life than it does in children. Because of this distinction, some people refer to this illness as "type 1.5 diabetes" informally. Based more on age than a cause, adults with LADA are often misdiagnosed as having type 2 diabetes at first. Adults with LADA produce more insulin than those with type 1 diabetes, but not enough to maintain normal blood sugar levels.

Meanwhile research initiatives related to diabetes are numerous and include both the hunt for treatments and the investigation of new technological frontiers

. While technical developments like artificial pancreas devices and closed-loop insulin delivery are reshaping the future of diabetes care, researchers are exploring a range of new treatments, including immune system modulation and beta cell regeneration.

Usually affecting adults more than children, type 2 diabetes is frequently linked to lifestyle choices. As a result Insulin resistance occurs in the body's cells, and the pancreas may find it difficult to generate enough of the hormone to meet the body's increased demand.

Elevated blood sugar levels are caused by both relative insulin insufficiency and insulin resistance. Although obesity, a poor diet, and inactivity can all increase the risk of Type 2 diabetes, these factors also have a major impact on the disease's development.

Type 2 diabetes is the most prevalent kind. . In nations of all income levels, the prevalence of type 2 diabetes has increased significantly during the last three decades, Type 2 diabetes accounts for approximately 90% of all instances of diabetes, with an anticipated 537 million individuals globally having the disease as of 2021, or 10.5% of adults. By 2045, nearly 783 million persons, or one in eight, are expected to have diabetes, a 46% rise from current estimates

Uncontrolled diabetes can cause major concerns due to elevated blood sugar levels, which can cause a variety of symptoms. Frequent signs and symptoms include thirst, weariness, impaired eyesight, and unexplained weight loss.

Changes in lifestyle, including a balanced diet, frequent exercise, and weight control, are often necessary for the management of diabetes. Blood sugar regulation may also involve the prescription of medications or insulin therapy. To effectively manage blood sugar and avoid complications including heart disease, renal difficulties, and nerve damage, regular monitoring of blood sugar levels is necessary.

Diabetes patients and healthcare providers frequently collaborate to create individualized treatment plans that meet each patient's unique needs and enable them to live long, healthy lives.

Causes And Risk Factors Of Diabetes Type 2

For the purpose of prevention, early detection, and efficient management, it is essential to comprehend the causes and risk factors of Type 2 diabetes. Here, we examine these important factors in greater detail:

*1. **Genetic Propensity**:

A major contributing factor to the development of Type 2 diabetes is genetics. People who have a family history of diabetes are more vulnerable. Insulin resistance, insulin production, and the general control of glucose metabolism can all be impacted by certain genetic variants.

2. **Body composition and obesity:**

Obesity is arguably the most powerful modifiable risk factor for Type 2 diabetes. An excess of body fat, especially visceral or abdominal fat, makes insulin resistance more likely. Hormones and inflammatory chemicals secreted by adipose tissue can obstruct the effects of insulin, raising blood sugar levels.

3. **Lack or little Body Exercise:**

It is commonly known that inactivity is a risk factor for Type 2 diabetes. Frequent exercise increases insulin sensitivity, which facilitates better glucose utilization by cells. Being inactive increases the likelihood of gaining weight and becoming obese.

4. **Unhealthy Food Practices**:

Diabetes risk is significantly influenced by dietary decisions. Diets heavy in sugars, saturated fats, and refined carbohydrates raise the risk of insulin resistance and obesity. On the other hand, diets high in fruits, vegetables, whole grains, and fiber have been linked to a decreased incidence of Type 2 diabetes.

5. Growing Older and Aging:

As people age, their risk of Type 2 diabetes rises. This is caused in part by the aging-related natural decrease in muscle mass and physical activity as well as the cumulative impact of lifestyle factors over time.

6. Diabetes during pregnancy:

Pregnant women who have gestational diabetes have a higher chance of subsequently getting Type 2 diabetes. Furthermore, there may be an increased risk of diabetes among offspring born to moms with gestational diabetes.

7. Race and Ethnicity:

Some racial and ethnic groups are more prone to Type 2 diabetes than others. Compared to people of European heritage, those of African, Hispanic, Native American, Asian, and Pacific Islander descent are more likely to get the illness.

8. **Resistance to Insulin:**

One of the main characteristics of Type 2 diabetes is insulin resistance. It happens when body cells lose their sensitivity to insulin's signals, especially muscle, liver, and fat cells. Consequently, there is inefficient absorption of glucose, which raises blood sugar levels.

9. **Hormonal Elements**:

Insulin resistance may be exacerbated by hormonal abnormalities. Type 2 diabetes is linked to conditions like polycystic ovarian syndrome (PCOS), which is characterized by anomalies in women's hormones.

10. **Hypertension, or elevated blood pressure:**

Type 2 diabetes has hypertension as a side effect and risk factor. Each condition exacerbates the other, and there is a reciprocal relationship between the two. Elevated blood pressure may result in arterial damage, which might impact the body's capacity to control glucose levels.

11. **Disorders of Sleep**: -

An essential component of metabolic health is sleep. Type 2 diabetes risk has been associated with chronic sleep loss and conditions including sleep apnea. Sleep disturbances can affect insulin control and other hormones.

12. **Stress and Mental Health**:

Long-term stress and mental health issues have been linked to the onset of Type 2 diabetes and insulin resistance. Blood sugar levels can rise as a result of stress hormones like cortisol interfering with insulin's ability to function.

13. **Smoking**:

Research has shown that one modifiable risk factor for Type 2 diabetes is cigarette smoking. Compounding the overall risk profile is smoking, which is linked to insulin resistance and an elevated risk of cardiovascular problems.

14. **Environmental Factors**:

Type 2 diabetes may arise as a result of environmental factors, such as exposure to specific chemicals and toxins. To learn more about the possible effects of environmental pollutants on metabolic health, research is still being done.

15. **Drugs and Medical Conditions**: -

Antipsychotics and corticosteroids are two examples of medications that may raise your risk of Type 2 diabetes. Diabetes risk can also be influenced by other illnesses such autoimmune disorders and cardiovascular disease.

Importance of Early Detection of Type 2 Diabetes

The diagnosis of Type 2 diabetes at an early age is essential to the overall healthcare strategy since it can significantly impact public health initiatives, optimize resource use in healthcare systems, and change individual health outcomes.

The substantial effects that prompt detection and action can have on people and society at large are highlighted by this complex significance. Meanwhile the capacity to enable prompt interventions for the best possible illness management is one of the most important advantages of early detection.

If left untreated, type 2 diabetes, which is frequently sneaky in its onset, can cause a host of other issues. Healthcare providers can start individualized management plans with early identification, which combine targeted pharmaceutical regimens and lifestyle changes based on each patient's unique needs. This not only attempts to delay or prevent issues from occurring, but it also greatly improves the quality of life for individuals who are dealing with this long-term illness.

One of the main principles of early detection is empowering people with knowledge. Being aware of one's personal risk factors for Type 2 diabetes promotes a proactive attitude and encourages active participation in preventive care and lifestyle modifications. A sense of control and agency over one's health is sparked by learning about the complex interactions that occur between nutrition, exercise, and stress reduction on blood sugar levels. People are encouraged to take an active role in their own well-being by being empowered, which serves as the cornerstone for long-term, maintained health.

The cornerstones of diabetes treatment include dietary changes, increased physical activity, and weight management. It is possible to incorporate these health-promoting behaviors into daily life with ease when Type 2 diabetes is identified and treated in its early stages. This helps to maintain overall health as well as help manage diabetes, which lessens the need for more extensive care when the condition worsens.

Additionally, stopping the progression from prediabetes—a condition that precedes Type 2 diabetes—is another reason why early detection is crucial. When people are diagnosed as prediabetic, it becomes easier to implement tailored therapies that emphasize dietary adjustments, weight loss, and increased physical activity

. In addition to demonstrating how early detection can change the trajectory of a disease, this preventative strategy highlights the transformative potential of lifestyle interventions in the field of public health. Also in terms of finances, early detection is consistent with the philosophy of efficient healthcare. Medical costs for complications, lost productivity, and emergency treatment are all included in the financial burden of diabetes.

By preventing or reducing the need for expensive hospital stays and treatments, prompt actions lessen these negative economic effects. Beyond personal concerns, the economic advantages take a broader perspective, relieving the financial burden on healthcare institutions and supporting a more sustainable approach to healthcare delivery.

A logical extension of early identification, individualized treatment plans emphasize how important it is to acknowledge the variability in how diabetes presents and reacts to care. Equipped with early detection, medical practitioners can create tailored treatment plans that maximize each person's results. By recognizing and adjusting to the particular nuances of every person's health journey, this customized approach goes beyond the limitations of a generic therapy strategy.

Early detection has implications that go beyond better resource management in healthcare systems. Early detection of Type 2 diabetes or those at risk for the disease allows for focused therapy, which reduces the need for emergency room visits or hospital stays brought on by uncontrolled diabetes. In a healthcare environment when resources are scarce, this not only optimizes resource allocation but also simplifies the delivery of healthcare.

Encouraging public health activities is evidence of the extensive influence of early detection. Public health initiatives can be refocused to address particular needs and challenges associated with Type 2 diabetes by identifying trends and risk factors within populations

. To achieve this, focused awareness campaigns, educational initiatives, and preventative strategies that are sensitive to the particular dynamics of different communities must be developed.

Essentially, early Type 2 diabetes identification becomes a complex, multimodal strategy that extends beyond personal health. It represents an approach to health that is proactive, fostering a culture of empowerment, preventive, and individualized care.

Early detection has cascade consequences that spread across society, making it a more resilient, knowledgeable, and health-conscious place to live. Early detection is a lighthouse that illuminates the way towards a future with better health outcomes and a sustainable, equitable healthcare paradigm as we traverse the intricacies of healthcare.

Kitty Carruthers, a national figure skating champion and Olympic medalist for the United States, did not let type 2 diabetes stop her from leading an active lifestyle. With the same determination that brought her success as an Olympic silver medalist (1984), a world bronze medalist (1982), and a four-time (1981–1984) United States national champion, she is committed to successfully maintain her health.

She stated, "Life lessons are what figure skating is all about." "It teaches you how to pick yourself up after falling." Kitty is adamant about leading a healthful life. She chuckled, "I'm lucky because I love good food."

Carruthers is driven to maintain her health so she may continue competing in sports and enjoy her family. She does admit that diabetes type 2 is a long-term condition. She remarked, "There are days when I watch other people eat cake and doughnuts." "I have a little pity party sometimes because life is unfair."

She is highly conscious of her health and feels that the only things she can do for herself are to eat healthily and exercise frequently. Carruthers has personal experience with the self-control needed for athletic success as a top athlete.

2. Meet Maria Rodriguez , one of my clients, and a 42-year-old marketing executive she visited for a check up. And upon receiving a type 2 diabetes diagnosis, found herself in a precarious situation. She claims no one in her family has ever had diabetes, and she is a very busy professional who rarely has time for healthy meals.

I had to give her professional advice and reassurance when I saw her at my office after assessing her situation, and together we came up with a comprehensive plan that included dietary adjustments, exercise regimens, and stress management techniques gotten through my years of expertise of practicing medicine, which have repeatedly worked all the same.

Maria, who had previously depended on quick but unhealthy meals, discovered a passion for cooking. She discovered a world of vibrant veggies, lean proteins, and whole grains under the nutritionist's tutelage. Maria found satisfaction in relishing meals that fed her body and used cooking as a therapeutic outlet.

Maria was required to work long hours at a desk due to her sedentary job. She thus received some quick, intense workouts that fit in perfectly with her hectic schedule. Maria's commute became an occasion to go on attentive walks around the neighborhood, and her lunch breaks turned into brisk walks.

Maria talked about her experience with her family and close friends. Her network of friends and family was, surprisingly, quite wide. Her dedication to wellness motivated her coworkers to start a group. After demanding workdays, they began planning stress-relieving potlucks, team exercise sessions, and even meditation sessions.

Maria's efforts paid off when her health began to improve many months into her quest. Weight loss, improved energy, and normalized blood sugar levels were all discovered during routine exams.After all, Type 2 diabetes is not always fatal; your ability to overcome it ultimately rests on your willingness and commitment.

Effectively controlling type 2 diabetes by can have a number of advantageous effects. The following are some possible advantages of managing type 2 diabetes well:

1. Decreased Complication Risk:

Diabetes consequences include cardiovascular disease, kidney problems, eye problems, and nerve damage can be reduced with proper management.

2. Improved Standard of Living:

Good management can enhance general wellbeing and enable people to have busy, meaningful lives.

3. Enhanced Vitality:

Maintaining steady blood sugar levels helps one feel energized all day long.

4. Improved Control of Weight:

A balanced diet and frequent exercise are important components of a healthy lifestyle that can help with weight management and even help with weight loss or maintenance.

5. Reduce Cholesterol and Blood Pressure:

Managing diabetes frequently entails lowering cholesterol and blood pressure, which lowers the risk of heart disease.

6. Preventing Low Blood Sugar:

Appropriate management lowers the chance of hypoglycemia-related problems by preventing episodes of low blood sugar.

7. Enhanced Mental Well-Being:

Effective diabetes management can improve mental health by lowering the stress, worry, and depression brought on by the illness.

8. Preventing Foot Problems Associated with Diabetes:

Infections and amputation risk can be decreased by managing or preventing foot issues with routine monitoring and care.

9. Improved Sleep:

Better sleep is a result of healthy living and stable blood sugar levels.

10. Decreased Inflammation:

A nutritious diet and regular exercise are two lifestyle modifications that may help lower inflammation in the body.

11. Reduced Chance of Further Health Problems:

Good diabetes control may improve general health and reduce the chance of developing additional chronic illnesses.

12. Enhanced Awareness and Self-Efficacy:

Understanding diabetes is a necessary part of managing the illness, and doing so can help people take charge of their health and make wise decisions.

13. Networks of Community and Support:

Developing a feeling of community and shared experience through connections with healthcare providers and support groups is a common aspect of managing diabetes.

CHAPTER 2

Diet plays a crucial role in the management and prevention of Type 2 diabetes, as it has a significant impact on these conditions. More than just a menu of options, diet is a dynamic factor that profoundly affects insulin sensitivity, blood sugar control, and general health. It is crucial for people, medical professionals, and public health initiatives to comprehend the complex relationship between nutrition and Type 2 diabetes.

However by treating nutrition as a comprehensive and individualized part of healthcare, it is possible to foster long-lasting, health-promoting habits that go beyond managing blood sugar levels to include general well-being. A very important factor in regulating blood glucose levels.

Foods high in carbohydrates, particularly refined sugars and highly processed carbs, can cause blood sugar levels to rise quickly. A diet high in complex carbs, including those found in whole grains, legumes, and vegetables, on the other hand, releases glucose more gradually and contributes to stable blood sugar levels.

Having a useful tool for creating diabetes-friendly diets called the glycemic index, which ranks foods according to how they affect blood sugar.

Apart from carbs, the kind and quantity of dietary lipids play a critical role in the context of Type 2 diabetes. Inflammation and insulin resistance may be exacerbated by saturated fats, which are frequently present in red meat and full-fat dairy products. As an alternative, including unsaturated fat sources like avocados, fatty salmon, and olive oil help reduce inflammation and improve insulin sensitivity.

Consuming enough protein is important as well, especially when it comes to meal preparation. Including foods high in lean protein, such fish, chicken, lentils, and tofu, can help control blood sugar levels and increase satiety. As part of balanced meals, protein should be distributed throughout the day to assist reduce post-meal glucose swings.

In order to effectively manage a Type 2 diabetic's diet, portion control and attentive eating are essential. Blood sugar and weight regulation can be achieved by regulating the amount of food consumed and paying attention to signals of hunger and fullness. This strategy puts more emphasis on creating a long-lasting and health-promoting relationship with food than it does on following rigorous diets.

The idea of eating patterns is becoming more important in the treatment of Type 2 diabetes than individual nutrients. Nutrition from a holistic perspective is emphasized by programs like the Dietary Approaches to Stop Hypertension (DASH) and the Mediterranean diet.

These eating patterns have an emphasis on whole, nutrient-dense diets that include a range of fruits, vegetables, whole grains, and lean meats. This all-encompassing method covers cardiovascular health as well as general well-being in addition to blood sugar control.

The effects of food decisions go beyond transient spikes in blood sugar. Long-term food choices have an impact on variables including body weight, which is a key component in the onset and course of Type 2 diabetes. The foundation of both diabetes prevention and control is the adoption of a diet that encourages weight management through a balance of energy intake and expenditure.

Dietary practices are significantly influenced by personal tastes and culture. When creating individualized nutrition regimens, it becomes crucial to acknowledge the diversity in dietary customs and preferences. Adapting dietary guidelines to cultural norms increases adherence and increases the likelihood that long-term dietary changes will be feasible.

Among the most important aspects of diabetes care are education and nutritional guidance. Giving people information about how their food choices affect their health makes it easier for them to make wise decisions. Making dietary decisions that support one's health objectives is made possible by knowledge of how various foods affect blood sugar levels.

In the larger framework of public health, encouraging a food environment that supports healthy choices and expanding access to nutrient-dense foods become crucial tactics. Diabetes prevention at the population level is aided by addressing "food deserts," areas where access to wholesome, fresh food is restricted, and by supporting legislative initiatives that promote better dietary options.

A balanced, well-rounded diet has an impact on more than just blood sugar regulation; it also affects weight management, metabolic health, and general well-being. Here, we examine the complex relationships between balanced diet and Type 2 diabetes.

1.Blood Sugar Regulation:-

Healthy fats, lean proteins, fiber, and complex carbs are all components of a balanced diet that help to keep blood sugar levels under control. Whole grains, fruits, and vegetables are rich sources of complex carbs, which release glucose gradually and reduce the risk of sharp surges. Plant-based foods contain fiber, which reduces the rate at which sugar is absorbed and helps to keep blood sugar levels steady. Proteins and lipids contribute to a balanced glycemic response during meals.

2. Insulin Sensivity;- Balanced nutrition has a good effect on insulin sensitivity, which is a major contributing factor to Type 2 diabetes. Insulin sensitivity is influenced by the kind and quality of carbs ingested. Improved insulin sensitivity is a result of diets that prioritize whole, unprocessed foods and reduce refined sugar intake. Improved insulin activity has been linked to healthy fats including those in nuts, avocados, and olive oil.

3. Weight control:

Retaining a healthy weight is essential for both controlling and avoiding Type 2 diabetes. Weight management is supported by a balanced diet that matches energy intake with energy expenditure. A sustainable strategy to weight control includes portion control, mindful eating, and selecting nutrient-dense foods. To increase insulin sensitivity, it is frequently advised for people with Type 2 diabetes to lose weight, if necessary.

4. Cardiovascular Health:-

Individuals who have Type 2 diabetes frequently have a higher risk of developing cardiovascular problems. Cardiovascular health is enhanced by a well-balanced diet, especially when it follows heart-healthy guidelines. Foods high in omega-3 fatty acids, which are present in whole grains, fruits, vegetables, and fatty fish like salmon, can lower cholesterol and lower the risk of cardiovascular problems.

5. Reduction of Inflammation: -

The development of Type 2 diabetes and insulin resistance are linked to chronic inflammation. Certain meals, like those high in anti-inflammatory lipids (found in olive oil and fatty fish) and antioxidants (found in fruits and vegetables), can help lessen inflammation. An anti-inflammatory environment in the body can be achieved with a balanced diet that emphasizes whole, nutrient-dense meals and reduces processed foods.

6. Micronutrient Support:-

Eating a balanced diet guarantees consuming the important vitamins and minerals required for good general health. Insulin sensitivity and glucose metabolism are influenced by micronutrients like magnesium, vitamin D, and antioxidants. These vital elements can be found in large quantities in a well-balanced diet that consists of a wide range of vibrant fruits and vegetables.

7. Constant Energy:-

Throughout the day, steady energy levels are facilitated by balanced eating. Meals containing a combination of carbohydrates, proteins, and fats help control how much energy is released. To prevent energy dips and maintain steady blood sugar levels, this is especially crucial for people with Type 2 diabetes.

8. Psychological Well-Being:-

It is important to consider the psychological effects of eating a balanced diet. Eating a balanced, diverse diet promotes a healthy relationship with food and eases the anxiety associated with preparing and consuming meals. A balanced diet can help maintain a general sense of vitality and resilience. Psychological well-being and physical health are linked.

9. Long-Term Disease Prevention:-

Eating a balanced diet contributes to both controlling current illnesses and preventing the onset of Type 2 diabetes. In addition to lowering the risk of developing insulin resistance and glucose dysregulation, healthy eating habits and an active lifestyle also support general metabolic health

Diabetes Type 2 And Carbohydrates Management

Managing carbohydrates is a crucial aspect of effectively controlling Type 2 diabetes. This dietary approach revolves around understanding the impact of different carbohydrates on blood sugar levels and making informed choices to maintain glucose stability. Instead of relying on rigid lists, managing carbohydrates involves a nuanced understanding of the quality, quantity, and timing of carbohydrate consumption.

Quality of carbohydrates is a fundamental consideration in this approach. Rather than labeling carbohydrates as "good" or "bad," the focus is on distinguishing between complex and refined carbohydrates. Whole grains, legumes, fruits, and vegetables provide complex carbohydrates that are rich in fiber. This fiber content slows down the absorption of glucose, preventing rapid spikes in blood sugar. On the other hand, refined carbohydrates, commonly found in sugary snacks and processed foods, can lead to quick increases in blood glucose levels.

Balanced meals that include a mix of carbohydrates, proteins, and fats are encouraged. This approach moves away from strict food lists and promotes variety and flexibility in dietary choices. Portion control becomes a key aspect of managing overall calorie intake and preventing large fluctuations in blood sugar levels.

Ways To Effectively Manage Your Carbohydrate Level

1. Individualized Approaches

Individualized approaches to carbohydrate management acknowledge the diverse needs, preferences, and cultural considerations of individuals with Type 2 diabetes. Instead of adhering to a universal set of dietary rules, healthcare professionals work with individuals to develop personalized plans that align with their lifestyle. This approach increases the likelihood of adherence and success in the long term.

2. Consistency and regularity

Consistency and regularity in meal timing and carbohydrate intake are emphasized. Irregular eating patterns or skipping meals can lead to unpredictable fluctuations in blood glucose levels. Establishing a routine that includes regular meals and snacks, distributed evenly throughout the day, helps maintain a more steady state of blood sugar.

3. Education And Empowerment

Education plays a central role in empowering individuals to make informed decisions about their diet. Understanding the nutritional composition of foods, interpreting food labels, and learning how different foods affect blood sugar levels are key components of this education. Armed with this knowledge, individuals can make choices that align with their health goals and contribute to effective diabetes management.

4. Monitoring And Adjusting

Monitoring blood sugar levels and adjusting dietary choices based on individual responses is an ongoing process. Rather than adhering strictly to a predetermined list, individuals can use real-time information about their blood sugar levels to make informed decisions about their diet. This iterative process allows for continuous refinement of dietary strategies.

5. Long Term Focus

A long-term focus is integral to carbohydrate management in Type 2 diabetes. It involves cultivating habits that promote overall well-being, including regular physical activity, stress management, and adequate sleep. This holistic approach recognizes the interconnected nature of various lifestyle factors in maintaining metabolic health and emphasizes sustainable, long-term habits rather than short-term fixes.

A sufficient intake of fiber in the diet is important for more reasons than only maintaining digestive health when managing Type 2 diabetes. Comprehending the complex influence of fiber on diverse facets of metabolic health highlights its indispensable function in advancing general health in individuals diagnosed with Type 2 diabetes.

1. Blood Sugar Regulation:

Dietary fiber has a significant impact on blood sugar levels, especially soluble fiber, which is present in foods like fruits, legumes, and oats. Soluble fiber slows down the digestion and absorption of carbs by forming a gel-like substance when it comes into contact with water. This process effectively prevents the fast blood sugar increases that can be harmful for people with Type 2 diabetes by causing a slow and controlled release of glucose into the bloodstream. To improve glycemic control, fiber's role in this area is crucial.

2. Insulin Sensitivity:

A key factor in the treatment of Type 2 diabetes is the correlation between increased insulin sensitivity and fiber consumption. Increased insulin sensitivity suggests that cells in the body react to insulin more efficiently, which helps to better control blood sugar levels. Given that insulin resistance is a major underlying problem in Type 2 diabetes, this effect is very important. Dietary fiber becomes an ally in the larger plan of treating the metabolic elements of the illness by encouraging increased insulin sensitivity.

3. Weight management:

Diets high in fiber promote feelings of fullness and satiety in addition to having a positive effect on blood sugar levels. Meals high in fiber frequently take longer to eat and involve more chewing, which encourages a slower pace of food consumption. This trait can result in a lower total caloric intake, helping people maintain a healthy weight or, if needed, reach weight loss objectives. Maintaining a healthy weight is essential for those with Type 2 diabetes since being overweight can make insulin resistance worse.

4 . Cardiovascular Health:

Since people with Type 2 diabetes may be more susceptible to heart-related problems, the cardiovascular advantages of fiber consumption are particularly significant for them. By attaching itself to cholesterol molecules, soluble fiber helps the body eliminate them. This procedure supports heart health by lowering LDL (low-density lipoprotein) cholesterol levels. Given the prevalence of cardiovascular issues associated with diabetes, the beneficial effects of fiber on cholesterol levels are especially noteworthy in this regard.

5. Stable Energy Release:

People with Type 2 diabetes benefit from fiber's ability to encourage a more steady and progressive release of energy from diet. Because of this trait, energy levels don't fluctuate during the day, which promotes mood stability and prolonged mental focus. Preventing energy crashes is crucial for general health and day-to-day functioning, which is consistent with the more general objective of holistic diabetes management.

6. Digestive Health:

Getting enough fiber in your diet is important for promoting digestive health, even though it has no direct bearing on blood sugar regulation. One of the benefits of a high-fiber diet is the avoidance of constipation and regular bowel movements. Furthermore, fiber contributes to a healthy gut flora, which benefits immune system and general gut health. For those with Type 2 diabetes, a healthy digestive tract is essential to their general comfort and well-being.

7. Variety in Nutrient Intake:

Foods high in fiber, like fruits, vegetables, whole grains, and legumes, are frequently high in nutrients. One can guarantee a varied intake of vital vitamins, minerals, and antioxidants by including a range of these items in their diet. This varied food profile supports the body's different metabolic processes and enhances general health. The way that fiber and other health-promoting ingredients work together in these foods emphasizes how crucial a comprehensive nutritional strategy is for managing diabetes.

Regular exercise and physical activity is an all-encompassing and effective approach to the fight against Type 2 diabetes. Exercise has a tremendous effect on many aspects of health, including insulin sensitivity, metabolic health, and general well-being. Here, we explore the many ways in which physical activity is essential for preventing and treating Type 2 diabetes.

1. Insulin Sensitivity

Exercise is a crucial factor in improving insulin sensitivity, which is important for managing Type 2 diabetes. Insulin sensitivity and glucose regulation are also improved by exercise. Regular exercise helps the body become more adept at using insulin, which makes it easier for cells to absorb glucose. Improved glucose management as a result of this increased sensitivity reduces the likelihood of insulin resistance, which is a major factor in the onset of Type 2 diabetes. The complicated connections between insulin-mediated glucose transport and exercise-induced physiological adaptations are the underlying mechanisms of this impact.

2. Weight management:

Exercise's ability to help people reach and maintain a healthy body weight is a key factor in its effects on Type 2 diabetes. Engaging in physical activity helps burn calories, which helps people who are overweight lose weight and keeps them from gaining it back. A balanced diet and regular exercise promote a long-term strategy to weight control. This is especially important because addressing a major factor in the development and progression of Type 2 diabetes depends on maintaining an ideal body weight.

3. Muscle Function and Health:

Exercise has a positive impact on the health and function of these vital tissues, which are essential for glucose metabolism. Muscles actively use blood glucose for energy when exercising, which promotes effective blood glucose absorption. Frequent exercise increases insulin sensitivity in the muscles and facilitates this process. Overall, this leads to a more efficient use of glucose, which significantly improves blood sugar regulation.

4. Cardiovascular Health:

Exercise is a powerful tool for promoting heart health, especially in light of the elevated cardiovascular risks linked to Type 2 diabetes. Exercise improves blood circulation, lowers blood pressure, and strengthens the heart—all important components of cardiovascular health. These cardiovascular advantages go beyond only lowering blood sugar levels right away; they also play a critical role in lowering the likelihood of cardiac problems associated with Type 2 diabetes.

5. Enhancement of Lipid Profile:

Physical activity leads to positive modifications in lipid profiles, which are crucial in attaining a more balanced concentration of triglycerides and cholesterol in the blood. Exercise helps to create a more desirable lipid profile by raising levels of high-density lipoprotein (HDL) cholesterol and lowering levels of triglycerides and low-density lipoprotein (LDL) cholesterol. This effect is especially important for controlling the increased cardiovascular risks that come with Type 2 diabetes.

6. Reducing Stress and Improving Mental Health:

Exercise's ability to reduce stress has consequences on metabolic and mental health. Exercise is a powerful stress-reduction strategy, and it has been shown that chronic stress is closely associated with insulin resistance. Physical activity causes endorphins to be released, which enhances mood and mental health. This beneficial psychological effect not only raises life quality overall but also develops a resilient mindset that is necessary to deal with the difficulties of having Type 2 diabetes.

1. Blood Pressure Regulation:

One of the most important aspects of total cardiovascular health is blood pressure regulation, which is greatly influenced by exercise. Engaging in regular physical activity helps lower high blood pressure, which lessens the burden on the heart and blood vessels. Given the connection between diabetes and cardiovascular problems, this regulation is very important and highlights the critical role exercise plays in the overall management of Type 2 diabetes.

2. **Better Sleep Patterns**:

Research has shown that consistent exercise is linked to better sleep. Sleep disturbances are associated with a higher risk of Type 2 diabetes, and enough sleep is essential for metabolic health. Exercise promotes improved overall sleep hygiene by helping to regulate sleep cycles. This higher-quality sleep further bolsters the physiological functions of the body that are involved in the metabolism of glucose.

It takes a deliberate, all-encompassing strategy to develop a fitness program that addresses the particular health problems associated with Type 2 diabetes.

Before starting any type of exercise program, people with Type 2 diabetes should consult with medical professionals such as an endocrinologist or their primary care physician. This holds especially true for assessing each person's health status, identifying potential risks, and receiving personalized guidance.

Recommended Exercises You Can Consider

1. Aerobic or Cardiovascular Activity:

Aerobic or cardiovascular exercise is essential for managing Type 2 diabetes. Attempt to complete at least 150 minutes per week of moderate-to-intense aerobic activity or 75 minutes of vigorous activity. Some of the activities include riding, swimming, walking quickly, and aerobic lessons. Benefits of cardiac exercises include improved insulin sensitivity, assistance with weight control, and overall cardiovascular health promotion.

2. Strength Training:

Try to fit in two days a week of strength training exercises. Focus on the major muscular areas of your body when using resistance bands, free weights, or weight machines. Strength training improves thermogenesis, increases lean muscle mass, and enhances overall functional fitness. Another benefit is that it regulates blood sugar.

3. Flexibility and stretching:

Perform stretches to improve joint strength and prevent injuries. Stretching before an exercise session and afterward with static stretches will help you become more flexible. Pilates and yoga are two types of exercises that increase flexibility and relaxation.

4. Balance Training:

Performing balance exercises is especially important for older adults with Type 2 diabetes. Methods for preventing falls and improving stability include using stability balls and performing difficult balance exercises, such as standing on one leg. Balance training is required for those with diabetic neuropathy.

1. Interval Training:

Consider doing interval training, which changes up the duration of your workouts by alternating short bursts of intense exercise with slower, more relaxed intervals. Due to its proven ability to raise insulin sensitivity more efficiently than continuous exercise, people with Type 2 diabetes can benefit from this method.

7. Regular Monitoring of Blood Sugar Levels: For diabetics using medicine or insulin, it's imperative to check blood sugar levels before and after exercise. This makes it easier to understand how different types and intensities of exercise impact blood sugar and to adjust medication or dietary intake as needed.

8.Customized Exercise Recommendation: Consider the different needs and capacities of individuals diagnosed with type 2 diabetes. Creating an exercise regimen should take into consideration each person's unique fitness level, interests, and any underlying medical conditions. A person with limited mobility or other diabetes-related concerns should have their needs adjusted.

9. Consistency and regular schedule:

Establish a regular, consistent fitness routine. Maintaining a regular exercise regimen is necessary to reap the long-term benefits of improved blood sugar management. Regulars help make exercise a habit and an essential part of everyday life.

10. Diet & Hydration:

Make sure you get enough water before, during, and after exercise. It is imperative for individuals with Type 2 diabetes to maintain a well-balanced diet that supports optimal energy levels and blood sugar regulation. Are you looking for customized dietary recommendations? Talk to a nutritionist who is licensed.

11. Increase Slowly and Steadily:

Gradually build up to a manageable level over time. Maintain physical health and refrain from overdoing it. Injury prevention is possible with steady advancement, as the body may adapt to increased physical activity.

12. Deep Breathing Exercises

Activities that lower stress, such as mindfulness meditation or deep breathing exercises, should be included in mind-body integration and stress reduction practices. Extended periods of stress can have an impact on blood sugar levels, and mind-body therapies enhance overall well-being.

13. Frequent Medical Check-ups:

Monitor your overall health and diabetes management with routine medical check-ups. The overall health benefits of exercise are highlighted by regular examinations that account for blood pressure, cholesterol, and other relevant indicators.

CHAPTER 3

A well-rounded and nourishing breakfast is crucial for those with Type 2 diabetes to help control blood sugar levels and provide them continuous energy throughout the morning. The following list of suggested breakfast ideas emphasizes complete, nutrient-dense foods:

Vegetable Omelette:

Ingredients: Eggs, spinach, onions, bell peppers, tomatoes, and feta cheese sprinkled on top.

Steps to prepare: beat eggs, transfer to hot pan with sautéed vegetables, and simmer until set. Once folded, serve.

Parfait with Greek Yogurt:

Greek yogurt, a handful of chopped nuts (almonds or walnuts), and berries (strawberries or blueberries) are the ingredients.

To make a tasty and high-protein breakfast, arrange Greek yogurt, berries, and almonds in a glass or dish.

A Chia Seed Oatmeal:

Almond milk, cinnamon, rolled oats, chia seeds, and fresh berries are the ingredients.

Prepare the ingredients for a satisfying and high-fiber breakfast by cooking the oats and chia seeds in almond milk, adding fresh berries, and topping with cinnamon.

Whole Grain Bread with Avocado Toast:

Ingredients: Optional cherry tomatoes, whole grain bread, ripe avocado, and a dash of salt & pepper.

To prepare, mash the avocado and spread it over a slice of whole grain toast. To enhance the taste, add cherry tomatoes, salt, and pepper.

Pineapple and cottage cheese:

Ingredients: pieces of fresh pineapple and cottage cheese.

Preparation: For a protein-packed and revitalizing breakfast, mix cottage cheese with pineapple.

Bowl of smoothies:

Combine spinach, kale, Greek yogurt, banana, and a few berries in a blender. Sprinkle granola, almonds, or seeds over top.

The smoothie can be prepared by pouring it into a bowl and adding your own toppings for a nutrient-rich breakfast.

Pancakes Made Whole Grain:

Ingredients include eggs, almond milk, whole wheat flour, baking powder, and a small amount of vanilla flavor.

To create whole grain pancakes, combine ingredients. Add some maple syrup or fresh berries on top.

The Chia Pudding

Ingredients: Almond milk, chia seeds, and a tiny bit of vanilla extract. Add raspberries or strawberries cut on top.

To prepare, blend almond milk, vanilla essence, and chia seeds. Refrigerate overnight, then top with berries the next morning.

Quinoa Breakfast Bowl:

Greek yogurt, cooked quinoa, chopped almonds, and honey drizzled over.

Prepare the dish by combining cooked quinoa, Greek yogurt, chopped almonds, and honey to create a high-protein breakfast bowl.

Whole Grain Toast with Cream Cheese and Smoked Salmon:

Smoked salmon, cream cheese, whole grain bread, and a dash of dill are the ingredients.

Breakfast can be made flavorful and filling by spreading cream cheese on whole grain toast, adding smoked salmon on top, and finishing with dill.

However always Keep an eye on portion amounts and think about speaking with a trained dietitian or healthcare provider to customize these breakfast options to your own dietary requirements and tastes.

Lunch And Dinner Recommendations To Combat Diabetes Type 2.

The following lunch and supper recipes highlight the importance of nutrient-dense, well-balanced meals to help people with Type 2 diabetes:

1. Salad with Grilled Chicken:

mixed greens, cucumbers, cherry tomatoes, and grilled chicken breast accompanied by a vinaigrette dressing.

Add avocado for additional fiber and good fats.

2. Bowl with quinoa and vegetables:

cooked quinoa, grilled shrimp or tofu, and sautéed veggies (zucchini, bell peppers, and broccoli).

For added taste, drizzle with olive oil and sprinkle with herbs.

3. Veggie and Turkey Wrap:

Lean turkey slices, lettuce, tomatoes, and hummus are all piled inside a whole wheat wrap.

Add some sliced cucumber or bell peppers for crispness.

4. Soup with Lentils:

Cooked lentil soup with spinach, carrots, and celery, flavored with a small pinch of cumin.

Serve with whole-grain crackers on the side.

5. Asparagus with Salmon:

Salmon fillet, baked or grilled, served with lemon wedges and roasted asparagus.

Serve with a little portion of sweet potatoes or quinoa.

Ideas for Dinner:

1. Roasted vegetables and baked chicken:

Brussels sprouts, cauliflower, and carrots are among the vibrant roasted veggies that go with baked chicken thighs.

Use herbs such as thyme and rosemary to season.

2. Tofu with Vegetables Stir-Fried:

Broccoli, bell peppers, and snap peas are among the vegetables stir-fried with tofu in a mild soy sauce.

Serve with cauliflower or brown rice on the side.

3. Grilled shrimp and zucchini noodles tossed with pesto:

grilled shrimp and homemade pesto atop zucchini noodles.

Basil, garlic, pine nuts, Parmesan cheese, and olive oil can all be used to make pesto.

4. Stir-fried veggies and beef:

Broccoli, mushrooms, and bell peppers are among the vibrant veggies stir-fried with lean beef strips in a low-sodium soy sauce.

Savor it with cauliflower rice or quinoa.

5. Curry with eggplant and chickpeas:

Curried eggplant and chickpeas with turmeric, coriander, and cumin in a tasty tomato-based curry sauce.

Serve with whole-grain flatbread or over quinoa.

6. Lemon and Herb Baked Cod:

Cod fillets cooked with lemon juice, olive oil, and a sprinkling of fresh herbs, such as dill or parsley.

Serve with a side salad or steaming green beans.

7. Tacos with cauliflower and chickpeas:

Whole-grain tortillas stuffed with taco-flavored roasted cauliflower and chickpeas.

Add some guacamole, salsa, and cilantro on top.

Overall Advice:

Portion Control: To control your consumption of carbohydrates, pay attention to portion sizes.

Consume a diet rich in fiber-rich foods, such as whole grains, legumes, and vegetables, to help control blood sugar levels.

Lean Proteins: Opt for foods high in lean protein, such as beans, fish, poultry, and tofu.

Healthy Fats: Include foods high in healthy fats, such as almonds, avocados, and olive oil.

Eat Fewer Processed Foods: Reduce the quantity of processed food, sugar-filled beverages, and refined carbs you consume.

For those with Type 2 diabetes, snack time is an opportunity to make healthy decisions that promote blood sugar control and general well-being. The following are things to look out for :-

1. Aim for a balance of the three macronutrients—carbohydrates, proteins, and fats—when preparing snacks. Long-lasting energy and blood sugar regulation are facilitated by this equilibrium. Apple slices with a little dollop of almond butter, for instance, mix carbohydrates with protein and healthy fats.

2. To prevent overindulging and keep your calorie intake consistent, it's important to practice portion management. Snack sizes can be modified to suit personal dietary requirements and tastes. Using small containers or measuring quantities can help you keep an eye on serving sizes.

3. Go for complete, minimally processed meals. Nuts, seeds, and fresh fruits and vegetables are great options. Without the additional sugars and bad fats that are frequently present in processed snacks, these

foods offer vital minerals, fiber, and antioxidants.

1. Fiber-rich Snacking:

Include high-fiber snacks since they assist reduce the rate at which sugar is absorbed and increase feelings of fullness. Fruits, vegetables, and whole grains are high in dietary fiber and provide a filling and healthy snack.

2. Options Packed with Protein:

Adding protein to snacks can help control blood sugar levels and enhance feelings of fullness. Good options include lean meats, Greek yogurt, cottage cheese, and plant-based protein sources like hummus or edamame.

Pay attention to your body's signals of hunger and fullness while you eat. Better digestion and an overall improved snacking experience can be achieved by eating mindfully, slowly, and appreciating flavors and sensations.

1. Hydration:

Take into account drinking water throughout snack time. Some great options are water, herbal drinks, or infused water with fruit or herb slices. For general health and to help manage cravings, it is important to drink enough water.

2. Low-Glycemic Snacks:

To reduce blood sugar rises, use low-glycemic snacks. Glycemic impact is typically reduced in foods like nuts, seeds, and non-starchy vegetables.

3. Snack Timing:

Take into account when to eat and when to exercise in relation to when you snack. While eating in between meals can help sustain consistent energy levels, overindulging in snacks is not advised, especially right before or right after meals.

Blood Sugar Monitoring:

Tracking blood sugar levels on a regular basis can reveal information about how various snacks influence people's reactions. Making educated decisions and changing snack alternatives requires knowledge of this information.

1. Customized Approach:

Understand that different people could react differently to different snacks. Adherence to a diabetes-friendly diet is improved by tailoring snack selections according to personal tastes, dietary constraints, and health objectives.

CHAPTER 5

Medication Management Of Diabetes
Type 2

Oral Treatment of Diabetes Type 2

It is noteworthy that the selection of oral drugs is contingent upon individual circumstances, including general health, kidney function, possible adverse effects, and responsiveness to the prescriptions. Maintaining a balanced diet and engaging in regular physical activity are other essential components of managing Type 2 diabetes.

An essential part of the treatment strategy for people with Type 2 diabetes is the use of oral medicines. These drugs are intended to help control blood sugar levels and enhance the body's reaction to insulin, the hormone that helps the body use glucose. The following describes the oral drugs that are often prescribed for Type 2 diabetes:

Metformin:

Mechanism of Action: The first-line drug metformin increases the body's sensitivity to insulin while lowering the amount of glucose produced in the liver.

Benefits: It lowers blood sugar levels during fasting and postprandial (after meals).

Take into account: For Type 2 diabetes, metformin is frequently administered as the first medicine. Although most people tolerate it well, some people may have gastrointestinal adverse effects.

Sulfonylureas:

Mechanism of Action: Sulfonylureas help to reduce blood sugar levels by stimulating the pancreas to release more insulin.

Advantages: They work well to reduce blood sugar, especially after meals.

Considering: Glipizide, glyburide, and glimepiride are examples of common sulfonylureas. Hypoglycemia, or low blood sugar, and weight gain are possible side effects.

DPP-4, or dipeptidyl peptidase IV, Restrictors:

DPP-4 inhibitors work by increasing insulin secretion and decreasing the liver's synthesis of glucose.

Advantages: Compared to some other drugs, they are generally well-tolerated and have a decreased risk of hypoglycemia.

Taking into account Sitagliptin, saxagliptin, and linagliptin are examples of common DPP-4 inhibitors.

TZDs, or thiazolidinediones:

Mechanism of Action: By increasing insulin sensitivity, TZDs facilitate the body's cells' improved utilization of insulin.

Advantages: They may be useful in lowering blood sugar and insulin resistance.

Take into account: Rosiglitazone and pioglitazone are common TZDs. Fluid retention and weight gain are possible side effects.

Glucosidase Inhibitors Alpha:

Mechanism of Action: These drugs lessen the amount of glucose absorbed by slowing down the intestinal breakdown of carbs.

Advantages: They assist in regulating blood sugar levels after meals.

Acarbose and miglitol are examples of common alpha-glucosidase inhibitors to take into consideration. Uncomfortable gastrointestinal side effects are possible.

Inhibitors of Sodium-Glucose Co-Transporter-2 (SGLT2):

Mechanism of Action: SGLT2 inhibitors increase the amount of glucose excreted in urine by decreasing the kidneys' ability to reabsorb glucose.

Advantages: They help with weight loss in addition to lowering blood sugar levels.

Notes: SGLT2 inhibitors that are often used include canagliflozin, dapagliflozin, and empagliflozin. Dehydration and a higher incidence of urinary tract infections are possible side effects.

When deciding which oral medicine regimen is best for each individual, medical professionals—such as endocrinologists and primary care physicians—have a critical role to play in taking into account their specific needs and circumstances. Effective diabetes management requires regular blood sugar testing and continuous communication with healthcare experts.

Insulin Therapy

When lifestyle changes and other drugs are not enough to achieve appropriate blood sugar control, insulin therapy is an option for treating Type 2 diabetes. Initially, oral drugs are commonly used to manage Type 2 diabetes. However, as the condition progresses, the body may become less capable of producing insulin or become more resistant to it. Insulin treatment becomes a useful tool in these situations to control blood sugar levels. For Type 2 diabetes, the following describes insulin therapy:

The list of indications for insulin therapy

1. **Insufficient Management of Blood Sugar**:

   When oral medications and lifestyle changes are made, the blood blood sugar levels persistently stay high.

2. When I'm Sick or Under Stress:

To guarantee the best possible blood sugar control, insulin therapy may be briefly started when sick or under stress.

3. To address various elements of blood sugar management, insulin may be given to oral drugs as part of combination therapy.

Insulin Types 2:

In order to address postprandial blood sugar rises, rapid-acting insulin is usually given shortly before meals. It acts swiftly.

1.Short-Acting (Regular) Insulin: Starts to function in 30 minutes and reaches its peak in 2-3 hours. 30 minutes before a meal is when it is often taken.

Insulin that functions as an intermediate between meals: It acts gradually and lasts for a longer period of time.

Insulin that acts as a background or basal insulin to keep blood sugar levels stable between meals and overnight is known as long-acting insulin. It releases insulin gradually over a prolonged period of time.

3. Insulin Delivery Methodologies:

Insulin pumps, pens, or syringes are used to provide insulin injections.

Insulin pumps allow for precise control by providing a constant supply of insulin through a tiny device worn on the body.

4. Insulin regimens

The basal-bolus regimen is a way to manage blood sugar rises by combining bolus insulin, which is administered before meals, with basal insulin, which acts as a long-acting insulin for background coverage.

Basal-Only Regimen: This plan, appropriate for certain people with fewer fluctuating blood sugar levels during meals, consists solely of long-acting insulin for background glucose control.

5. Dosage and Timing:

Individualized Approach: The administration of insulin therapy is highly customized, with dose determined by blood sugar levels, lifestyle choices, and eating habits, including diet.

Titration: In order to attain the best blood sugar control, insulin dosages are gradually modified.

6. Monitoring and safety:

Accurately determining the efficacy of insulin therapy and adjusting dosages require routine blood sugar monitoring.

Hypoglycemia Management: Insulin users need to be aware of the signs of low blood sugar, or hypoglycemia, and know how to treat it right away.

7. Education and assistance:

Those on insulin therapy require instruction on how to inject correctly, store insulin, and check their own blood sugar levels.

Diabetes Management Support: Insulin therapy success depends on ongoing assistance from medical professionals, diabetes educators, and support groups.

8. Lifestyle Factors: Diet: Important aspects of insulin therapy include meal preparation and carb counting.

Exercise: Consistent exercise has the potential to affect insulin sensitivity and insulin therapy efficacy.

9. Potential Advantages:

Better Blood Sugar Control: Insulin treatment aids in lowering blood sugar levels to within the desired range.

Flexibility: To suit varying lives and interests, various insulin kinds and regimens offer flexibility.

10. Special Populations:

A Few Points to   Remember

Older People: Dependent on variables including kidney function and general health, insulin dosage may need to be adjusted.

Women Ahead: To control blood sugar levels and lower the risk of problems during pregnancy, insulin therapy is frequently utilized.

Chapter 6

An essential part of treating Type 2 diabetes is keeping an eye on blood sugar levels. In addition to helping people make educated decisions about changing their lifestyles and taking medications, regular monitoring gives important information about how well the treatment plan is working and helps healthcare providers optimize the management of diabetes. The purpose of blood sugar monitoring for Type 2 diabetes is explained as follows:

Objective of Blood Sugar Monitoring:

Blood sugar levels are assessed by monitoring, which enables people to comprehend their present blood sugar levels, including postprandial levels following meals and fasting levels in the morning.

Modification of Treatment:

In order to attain ideal blood sugar regulation, the results inform modifications to drug dosages, way of life decisions, and food habits.

A regular monitoring schedule aids in the identification of trends and patterns that, if left unchecked, may lead to difficulties.

2. **Blood Sugar Test Types**:

Going without food A blood sugar test is performed, usually before morning, to determine blood sugar levels following an overnight fast.

Blood sugar levels are measured 1-2 hours after a meal using the postprandial blood sugar test, which determines how food affects glucose levels.

An extended view of glycemic management is provided by the HbA1c test, which yields the average blood sugar levels over the previous two to three months.

1. Frequency of Monitoring:

Individualized Approach: Individualized blood sugar monitoring differs from person to person and is frequently influenced by a variety of circumstances, including personal preferences, treatment plans, medication schedules, and general health.

2. .Intensive Management:

Regular monitoring, especially before and after meals, may be necessary for patients on insulin therapy or with more complicated treatment regimens.

3. Blood glucose meters:

Blood glucose monitoring at home: Using a tiny drop of blood drawn from a finger prick, portable blood glucose meters enable people to check their blood sugar levels at home.

Some people may utilize continuous glucose monitoring (CGM) devices, which give them real-time information on their blood sugar levels all day long. A broader perspective on glucose swings may be provided by CGM devices.

Interpreting Blood Sugar Readings: Target Ranges: Individuals collaborate with healthcare professionals to determine target blood sugar ranges for HbA1c, postprandial, and fasting conditions.

Hyperglycemia: Appropriate treatment may be indicated by elevated blood sugar levels, necessitating changes in medicine or way of life.

Hypoglycemia: When taking some medications, low blood sugar might happen. This condition may need to be treated right away to avoid problems.

6. **Maintaining Documents**: Blood Sugar Records: Both patients and medical professionals can benefit greatly from keeping a detailed record of blood sugar readings, meals, prescriptions, and activities.

Technology Integration: To facilitate the recording and sharing of data, a number of blood glucose meters and continuous glucose monitoring (CGM) devices can sync with computers or cellphones.

7. **Treatment Plan Modifications:** Medication Modifications: Healthcare professionals may suggest new medication or adjustments to dosage in order to maximize control based on blood sugar readings.

Adjustments to Lifestyle: Dietary choices, physical activity, and stress management are all guided by blood sugar monitoring.

8. Consulting with healthcare providers and conducting routine follow-ups Treatment plan modifications and continuous evaluations are ensured by routine follow-ups with healthcare professionals, such as diabetes educators, endocrinologists, and primary care physicians.

9. Empowerment and Education:

Patient education helps people comprehend how to interpret blood sugar levels, grasp the effects of lifestyle decisions, and spot the warning symptoms of hypo- or hyperglycemia.

Self-Management:

It is possible for people to actively control their diabetes when they are aware of how daily decisions impact blood sugar levels.

Personalization:

Adaptability on an Individual Basis Individual variations in blood sugar levels are common. There is heterogeneity in this regard due to several factors like age, general health, comorbid illnesses, and individual reaction to medicine.

1. The goal of blood sugar monitoring is to evaluate control. Frequent monitoring aids in assessing the effectiveness of blood sugar regulation throughout the day, including readings during fasting and after meals.

Treatment Modifications:

Based on the data acquired from monitoring, medical professionals can alter the dosage of insulin, medicines, and other elements of the treatment regimen.

2. Keeping consequences at Bay: Maintaining stable blood sugar levels lowers the chance of developing long-term diabetes-related consequences like kidney disease, nerve damage, and heart disease.

Techniques for Tracking Blood Sugar:

Blood glucose meters are carry-along gadgets that let people check their blood sugar levels at home using a tiny drop of blood, usually drawn from a fingerstick.

Continuous glucose monitoring (CGM): A real-time data and trend-tracking device that measures blood glucose levels constantly day and night.

3. How Frequently You Monitor:

Fasting Blood Sugar: This is usually checked first thing in the morning, before any food or liquids are consumed. It offers a blood sugar baseline.

Postprandial Blood Sugar: Measured following meals to determine how dietary decisions affect blood sugar levels.

Random Blood Sugar: Measured throughout the day to assess blood sugar levels at various periods.

4. Goal Blood Sugar Levels:

 Fasting Blood Sugar: The aim is normally within the range of 70 and 130 mg/dL.

After meals, blood sugar levels should be kept below 180 mg/dL, though specific targets may differ.

HbA1c: This test gives you the average blood sugar reading for the previous two to three months. Usually, the goal is less than 7%.

5. Interpreting Blood Sugar Readings:

Hypoglycemia (Low Blood Sugar): If the readings are less than the desired range, it may be hypoglycemia. Sweating, agitation, disorientation, and shakiness are some of the symptoms.

Hyperglycemia, or high blood sugar, can be indicated by readings that are higher above the recommended range. Increased thirst, frequent urination, exhaustion, and impaired vision are among the symptoms.

6. Blood Sugar-Related Factors:

Blood sugar levels can be greatly impacted by the kind and quantity of carbohydrates ingested, as well as the timing of meals.

Physical Activity:

Depending on its length and intensity, exercise can either raise or drop blood sugar levels.

Medicines:

Blood sugar control is influenced by adherence to medication regimens, which include insulin or oral medicines.

7. Continuous Glucose Monitoring (CGM):

Real-Time Data: CGM devices give users access to continuous, real-time data on their blood sugar levels, providing a thorough understanding of variations.

Alerts and Trends: Continuous glucose meters (CGMs) can notify users of possible high or low blood sugar levels and offer insights into long-term trends.

2. Record-Keeping:

Diabetes Logbook: Individuals and healthcare professionals can see trends and make well-informed decisions by keeping a journal of their blood sugar readings, meals, and physical activity.

Digital applications: A lot of people use applications for managing their diabetes, which let them record and monitor their blood sugar levels, meals, and other pertinent data.

9. Routine Medical Exams:

HbA1c Evaluation: This blood test, which is performed every two to three months, gives an average of the blood sugar levels throughout time.

Medical Reviews: Routine check-ups with healthcare professionals enable a thorough assessment of blood sugar regulation and general health.

10. **Patient Education**: Interpreting Results: People with Type 2 diabetes need to be taught how to read their blood sugar levels and comprehend the implications for their overall care.

Troubleshooting: For efficient self-management, knowledge of how to troubleshoot high or low blood sugar levels is crucial.

Diabetes type 2 can affect the macrovascular (bigger blood vessels) and microvascular (smaller blood vessels) systems in the blood circulation. Additional problems and impacts of type 2 diabetes that affect blood circulation are listed below:

1. Aged Hands or Feet:

Feeling cold in the hands and feet can be caused by reduced blood supply to the extremities, even in warm weather.

2. Issues with the feet:

Diabetes-related foot issues can be a sign of poor circulation and nerve damage. These issues include ulcers, infections, and deformities.

3. Aches in the Legs or Feet, Particularly at Night:

People with diabetes who also have impaired circulation may feel pain or discomfort in their legs and feet, especially at night.

4. Diminished Feeling:

Reduced feeling in the extremities may be the result of nerve injury. There's a chance that people won't notice injuries because they won't experience heat, cold, or pain as strongly.Pain in the Legs When Walking

5. Claudication

A condition when there is insufficient blood flow to the legs, can hurt or cramp when exercising. Resting often helps with this.

6. Shaving of the Lower Extremities Hair:

Inadequate blood flow can damage hair follicles, resulting in hair loss on the feet and lower legs.

7. Enamel thickening or discoloration:

The thickening or yellowing of toenails, or other changes in their texture and color, may be a sign of impaired circulation.

8. The insufficiency of veins

Venous insufficiency is a disorder in which the veins have trouble pumping blood from the legs to the heart. Diabetes can aggravate this problem. Ulcers, discomfort, and edema may follow from this.

9. Abnormalities of Blood Clotting:

Blood clot development may be more likely in those with diabetes. Blood channel blockages caused by clots can result in consequences including deep vein thrombosis (DVT) or pulmonary embolism.

10. Enhanced Inflammation

Diabetes-related chronic inflammation can exacerbate vascular deterioration and poor blood flow.

11. Neuropathy of the Autonomic Nervous System:

Blood vessel function-regulating nerves may be impacted by autonomic neuropathy, a kind of nerve disease that is frequently associated with diabetes. This may result in issues controlling blood pressure and impairing general circulatory health.

12. Decreased Movement of Collateral:

The network of smaller blood vessels known as collateral circulation, which might offer backup blood flow channels in the event of blockages, may be impacted by diabetes.

13. Impaired Healing of Wounds:

Wound healing may be slowed down by diabetes-related poor blood circulation. Decreased blood flow makes it more difficult for immune cells and nutrients that are essential for healing to reach the body.

14. Reduced Sulfur Oxide Production:

Vasodilators like nitric oxide aid in the relaxation of blood vessels. Diabetes may lower the synthesis of nitric oxide, which can lead to vasoconstriction and poor blood flow.

15. Higher Chance of Infections:

The body's defenses against infections can be weakened by poor circulation, especially in the extremities. This can increase the risk of foot infections and problems in those with diabetes.

16. Gangrene:

Gangrene can develop in extreme situations of impaired circulation, particularly when it is exacerbated by an infection. This medical emergency is caused by the death of bodily tissue.

17. Anguish or Unease in the Calves:

People who have diabetes and poor circulation may feel pain or discomfort in their calves, particularly when they exercise. This may indicate that the blood supply to the leg muscles is diminished.

18. Exuberant or taut skin:

Reduced elasticity, which can be brought on by inadequate circulation, can make the skin on the lower extremities seem tight or shiny.

Type 2 diabetes and its effect on blood circulation is massive , consider these methods to possibly improve blood circulation : Always get your healthcare team's approval before making any big adjustments

1. Add Foods High in Nitrates to Your Diet:

Foods high in nitrates, such celery, beets, and leafy greens (arugula, spinach), help improve blood circulation. The body uses nitrates to produce nitric oxide, which improves blood flow and vasodilation.

2. Examine hydrotherapy:

During a shower or bath, switching between hot and cold water might help to promote blood circulation. You can achieve this by briefly switching between warm and cold water.

3. Examine supplements containing ginkgo biloba:

A natural supplement called ginkgo biloba may have vasodilatory effects and enhance blood circulation. But you should talk to your healthcare physician about using it.

4. Practice Breathing Mindfully:

Deep diaphragmatic breathing is one mindful breathing technique that might help relax blood vessels and enhance circulation. Incorporate these daily habits in your everyday life.

5. Investigate acupressure or acupuncture:

Acupuncture and other traditional Chinese medicine techniques like acupuncture may be taken into consideration to enhance circulation. See a trained professional for individual guidance.

6. Put on compression clothing:

Wearing compression sleeves or stockings can help to improve blood circulation, especially in the legs. Find out if this is right for you by speaking with your medical team.

7. Include Foods High in Fatty Acids (Omega-3:

Fish, flaxseeds, and chia seeds are rich sources of omega-3 fatty acids, which may offer anti-inflammatory properties that improve blood circulation and cardiovascular health.

8. Examine Biofeedback Methods:

Using electronic monitoring to acquire awareness and control over body functions, biofeedback techniques have the potential to improve blood flow and assist manage stress.

9. Employ Electrolytes to Remain Hydrated:

Blood circulation depends on enough hydration. Make sure you drink enough water, and for best balance, think about consuming electrolyte-rich beverages as well

10. Examine Herbal Teas:

It is thought that some herbal teas, such ginger tea and hawthorn tea, may be good for cardiovascular health. It is best to speak with your healthcare practitioner before starting any new regimen.

11. Use Vibration Therapy for the Whole Body:

Standing on a vibrating platform can provide whole-body vibration, which has the potential to increase muscular tone and blood flow. A healthcare expert should provide instruction when performing this.

12. Do Tai Chi or Yoga

Mind-body practices, such as tai chi or yoga, have the ability to improve blood circulation, lessen tension, and encourage relaxation. Select workouts based on your preferences and level of fitness.

13. Massage Therapy:

A massage may ease tension, enhance blood flow, and relax muscles. Speak with a licensed massage therapist and let them know you have diabetes.

14. Think About Supplements with Herbs:

Certain herbal supplements, such as bilberry or horse chestnut extract, may be beneficial for blood circulation. However, you should talk to your healthcare practitioner about their efficacy and safety.

15. Limit your prolonged sitting:

Poor blood circulation can be exacerbated by prolonged sitting. Incorporate standing, stretching, and movement breaks into your daily routine, particularly if you work a sedentary job. Consult your healthcare provider before making any big changes. With type 2 diabetes, consider these lesser-known methods to possibly improve blood circulation

16. Give up smoking.

The risk of cardiovascular issues, which can ultimately impede blood flow, is elevated by smoking. It would benefit your circulatory system more if you can quit smoking as soon as possible.

CHAPTER 7

Controlling Diabetes Type 2 With Stress Management

For people with Type 2 diabetes, managing stress is essential since it can impact blood sugar levels and general health. Prolonged stress can cause alterations in lifestyle choices, like poor dietary habits and less exercise, which can make managing diabetes more difficult. The following explains how to manage stress in the context of type 2 diabetes:

1. Identifying Stress:

 Physical Symptoms: Stress can cause physical symptoms such headaches, tense muscles, and digestive problems.

Emotional Signs: Common emotional reactions to stress include increased irritability, mood fluctuations, anxiety, and feelings of overload.

2. Recognizing the Link Between Stress and Diabetes:

Cortisol production: Stress causes the production of stress hormones, including cortisol, which can raise blood sugar levels.

Impact on Behavior: Stress can affect lifestyle choices like overindulging in food or choosing less healthful foods, which can affect blood sugar regulation.

3. **Strategies for Reducing Stress**:

Deep breathing exercises and mindfulness meditation are two techniques that can help reduce tension and encourage relaxation.

Physical Activity: Engaging in regular exercise helps to lower stress levels. Endorphins are released as a result, and they naturally elevate mood.

Hobbies: Taking part in pleasant activities can help you feel fulfilled and accomplished while also serving as a stress reliever.

4. **Time Management**:

Task Prioritization: You can feel less overwhelmed by dividing activities into smaller, more manageable steps and setting them in order of importance.

Setting Boundaries: Burnout and undue stress can be avoided by clearly defining boundaries for work and personal time.

4. Social Support:

Making Connections: Talking to friends, relatives, or support groups about how you're feeling might help you get perspective and emotional support.

Expert Assistance: Seeking guidance from mental health specialists, such psychologists or counselors, can provide customized approaches to managing stress.

5. Healthy Lifestyle Options:

Balanced Diet: Eating a nutritious, well-balanced diet promotes general health and helps to stabilize blood sugar levels.

Sufficient Sleep: Make high quality sleep a priority because it greatly affects stress levels and general health.

Reducing Stimulants: Since stimulants like caffeine can exacerbate tension and anxiety, cut back on your intake of these substances.

7. Behavioral-Cognitive Methods:

Restructuring cognition: It can be beneficial to recognize and confront negative thought patterns in order to alter one's perspective of stresses.

Problem-Solving: Having strong problem-solving abilities might enable people to deal with stress in a positive way.

8. **Consistent Diabetes Care**: Following the Treatment Plan: Maintaining control even during stressful times can be achieved by faithfully adhering to the diabetic treatment plan, which includes taking medicine, checking blood sugar levels, and scheduling doctor's appointments.

Flexibility in Meal Planning: Having flexible meal planning might help lessen the impact on blood sugar levels by acknowledging that stress may affect eating habits.

Goal Setting:

Realistic Expectations: Stress related to perceived expectations can be reduced by setting realistic objectives and recognizing accomplishments of any size.

Dividing Larger chores into Manageable phases: You can reduce the sense of overwhelm by dividing larger chores into smaller, more manageable phases.

10. **Mind-Body Techniques**: Biofeedback and Relaxation Methods: Using biofeedback or

relaxation techniques, one can learn to regulate one's body's physiological reactions to stress.

Visualization: Turning your mind from stressful situations to peaceful, upbeat ones can assist.

11. **Consistent Self-Evaluation**: Examining Stressors: Stress management techniques can be continuously adjusted by analyzing coping mechanisms and stress causes on a regular basis.

12. **Expert Advice**:

 Counseling Medical Group: Healthcare professionals can provide individualized recommendations that support diabetes treatment objectives by talking about stress management techniques.

Chapter 8

Building A Support System to Combat Type 2 Diabetes

For those with Type 2 diabetes, developing a strong support network is essential. Having a strong support network can help with diabetes control and general well-being by offering emotional support, useful help, and understanding. An in-depth conversation about the significance of creating a support network for people with Type 2 diabetes can be found here:

1. **Emotional Assistance**:

Knowledge and Compassion: A network of support is aware of the emotional and practical difficulties associated with having diabetes. A sympathetic friend or relative can provide emotional support and a listening ear.

Mental Health: Managing diabetes can be emotionally draining. People who have a support network find it easier to manage stress, worry, and depression—common problems linked to long-term illnesses.

2. **Useful Help**: Meal Planning and Preparation: Caring people can help with the planning and preparation of wholesome meals that follow diabetic dietary requirements.

Physical Activity: It can be motivational to encourage regular exercise and engagement in physical activities. Activities might be enhanced by the participation of a buddy or supportive partner.

3. **Education and Awareness**: Type 2 Diabetes Education: Creating a network of support requires informing those in close proximity about the symptoms, causes, and possible obstacles of Type 2 diabetes. Informed support and understanding are fostered by this shared knowledge.

Going to medical appointments with a supportive companion can help ensure that patients fully comprehend the instructions and treatment plans provided by their healthcare providers.

4. **Communication and Open Dialogue**: • **Open Communication**: When channels of communication are established, people can freely express their demands, worries, and

emotions. A supportive atmosphere requires effective communication.

Collaborative decision-making is promoted when supportive individuals are included in decisions about treatment alternatives, lifestyle modifications, and day-to-day care.

5. **Encouraging Healthy Habits**:

 Positive Reinforcement: Having a supportive network can help you adopt and stick to healthy lifestyle practices including getting enough sleep, exercising on a regular basis, and eating a balanced diet.

Honoring Accomplishments: Highlighting and commemorating accomplishments, no matter how minor, fosters a good and inspiring environment.

6. **Problem-Solving and Coping Strategies**:
Brainstorming Solutions: When confronted with obstacles in the management of diabetes, a support system can hold brainstorming sessions in order to identify workable solutions.

Coping methods: People who are supportive can help others create and use efficient coping methods to deal with stress, frustration, and setbacks.

7. **Inclusion in Social Activities**: Fostering a Supportive Social Environment: Friends and family can help foster a social environment that is sensitive to the requirements of people managing their diabetes. For instance, selecting health-conscious dining establishments or incorporating exercise into social events.

Recognizing Limitations: A caring support system acknowledges and acknowledges the constraints placed on a person with diabetes without making them feel alone.

8. **Joint Accountability**: Family and Home Assistance: Meal planning, grocery shopping, and setting up a diabetic-friendly environment at home are some of the duties associated with controlling diabetes. Working together to complete these activities promotes a sense of collaboration.

Emergency Preparedness: A supporting network can receive training on what to do in case of low blood sugar or other diabetes-related emergency, including emergency protocols.

9. **Online and Community Support**:

Virtual Support Groups: These online communities and support groups offer a forum for interacting with people going through comparable experiences. Exchanging insights and advice might be beneficial.

Community activities: Participating in diabetes-related activities and support groups in the area offers chances to expand one's support system.

10. **Caregiver Involvement**: Caregivers are essential to the daily lives of those with diabetes because they help with medication management, everyday support, and medical treatment.

Opportunities for respite and having their own support network are beneficial for caregivers as well.

11. **Professional Assistance**:

Medical Staff: An integral component of the support network is the medical staff, which consists of physicians, diabetes educators, and nutritionists. Effective diabetes control involves regular check-ins and engagement with medical specialists.

Advocacy and Awareness: Promoting Individual Advocacy Those with diabetes who have a strong support system can serve as advocates, guiding them through social settings, professional environments, and healthcare facilities.

Increasing Diabetes Awareness: Friends and relatives can help spread knowledge and compassion about diabetes throughout the community.

Within "Snuff Out Diabetes Type 2," we've taken an enlightening journey through a lot of techniques and principles for to attain complete freedom .

As we come to an end of this investigation, it is evident that living with and even beating type 2 diabetes requires a significant transformation of resilience, mindset, and way of life. Obviously seming like a complex dance between dedication, understanding, and the steadfast support of a community.

 It's an appeal to readers to reevaluate how they relate to their health and welcome the prospect of positive change.

The general idea of this book focuses on the fact that that type 2 diabetes need not be a death sentence but rather a turning point toward a healthier, more energetic life. This story goes beyond the confines of a specific illness, inspiring us to see the connections between the decisions we make, the resiliency we possess, and the significant impact of our community.

many people dealing with type 2 diabetes find direction, strengthen their ability to accept change, foster a community of support, and set out on a path to long-term wellness.

. Cheers to you, health, resiliency, and all the opportunities ahead as you continue on your unique journey to overcome type 2 diabetes.

www.ingramcontent.com/pod-product-compliance
Lightning Source LLC
Chambersburg PA
CBHW070953250726
48663CB00002B/201